Menopause and Your Career

Strength in the Storm - Working Woman's Guide to Menopause in the Workplace

Alex Locklear

Table of content:

Introduction:

Ladies, let's be honest. Menopause is like having a crazy aunt who shows up out of the blue, stays too long, and washes your whole life in hormones. My trip? That's like having hot flashes, brain fog as thick as pea soup, and mood swings that are harder to predict than a teenager while trying to do a hard job. I might be fanning myself in secret during a board meeting, fighting the urge to cry during a presentation, or forgetting the name of a client in the middle of a statement. It looked bad.

At first, I thought I was the only one going through this. When I saw women in the office who were calm and professional, I felt ashamed. Why did I lose it? It got worse because no one talked about menopause. I was too ashamed to ask for help, but I was drowning in sweat, worry, and self-doubt. Not until I told a few trusted coworkers what was bothering me did the weight start to lift. According to what they said, they were fighting their own menopausal problems. It felt great to talk about it.

That's why this book is important. Millions of women go through menopause at work, but it's kept secret and looked down upon. The message that we should "power through" sticks with us, even though our bodies and minds are fighting against it. The thing is, we don't have to suffer in silence. It's time to break the rules, ask for help, and speak up for ourselves. This book isn't just about how to handle this crazy ride; it's also about changing the rules and taking back our power at work, menopause and all.

Why We Should Talk About It Now

It's finally being seen what the elephant in the corner office is. Women at work have been whispering about menopause in the bathroom for years, and it's been a worry in the back of our minds. But things are changing, and it's a good thing. This talk is more important than ever because:

• The Facts Are True: Women who have gone through menopause are the fastest-growing group in the workforce. What we are is not a small group; we are a powerful force. Ignoring this fact is just bad business.

• Less work gets done: menopause symptoms aren't just a bother; they can really mess up your work life. There are huge hidden costs for companies (and our jobs) when we miss deadlines or don't show up for work.

• Caring for your mental health: People who are going through menopause often also have anxiety, sadness, and burnout. Employees are healthier and more involved when they can talk to each other freely and get help at work.

• A New Generation Speaks Out: Unlike groups before us, who often went through menopause alone, we want a more understanding approach. We want places of work that understand what we need and can help us find it.

You're Not By Yourself: Finding Help in a Problem We All Face As bad as the hot flashes can be, being alone during menopause can be even worse. We think we're the only ones having a hard time, but a lot of other women are going through the same thing. Getting out of isolation is important for our health and our ability to push for change. How to find your tribe:

• The Power of Supporting Each Other: It feels great to talk to other women at work who understand what you're going through. Find people you trust, or think about starting a small, private menopause support group at lunchtime.

• The growth of online communities: Women talk about all aspects of menopause online, including the good, the bad, and the funny. There are Facebook groups and sites just for this purpose. Connect with other women online and share without feeling bad about it.

• Don't forget how important family and friends are: Your partner might not fully understand what you're going through with brain fog, but having someone to talk to and lean on is very helpful. Tell the people closest to you things that are bothering you so they can help you.

Advocacy Begins with You: Taking Responsibility for Your Story Workplaces that are friendly to women going through the menopause are important, but the most important change we can make is within ourselves. It's about taking responsibility for our experience, standing up for our wants, and not putting up with a system that wasn't made with us in mind. In other words:

Of course! Building on what we've already said, here's what comes next:

• Letting Go of the Shame: Our worst enemy is internalized shame. It says that our problems are "weak" or "unprofessional." Start arguing against those harmful ideas. Menopause is a normal part of life, not a sign of a bad person.

• Getting to Know Yourself: It's true that knowledge is power. Learn about the signs of menopause, the different ways to treat it, and your rights as an employee. Being able to speak up for yourself with more confidence comes from knowing more about the subject.

• Getting used to having tough conversations: It can be scary to talk to your boss or HR about menopause. Play the part with a friend and write down important points. Keep in mind that you're asking for fair adjustments that will help both you and the company.

• Know Your Worth: Don't let going through menopause make you doubt yourself. Your boss needs the skills and knowledge you have to offer. You should look into your options if you don't feel supported. It could be a different job at work or a whole new environment.

What the Challenge and the Chance Are

Let's not sugarcoat it: pushing for menopause at work won't be easy. We have to deal with old ideas, lack of knowledge, and sometimes outright bias. Let's change the story, though: this is also a huge chance. For our own sake, the sake of our female coworkers, and for the sake of the generations that will come after us at work. When we speak out, we show that everyone is welcome. When we ask for help, we push for laws that take into account how women's bodies really are and give us room to thrive at all stages of life.

Also, it doesn't hurt to laugh sometimes, especially when you're going through the crazy things that come with menopause. Let's laugh at the hot flashes, talk about the embarrassing times, and celebrate how strong we are when our hormones change. Don't forget that we're all in this together. By speaking out, helping each other, and taking pride in our strength, we can make it so that menopause is no longer a taboo subject at work but a normal part of a woman's life that is accepted and celebrated.

What Will Happen Next?

Well, reading this book is already a big step in the right direction. It's not enough to just read; you have to do something. We will talk about all the specifics of menopause and the job along the way. We'll talk about the science behind those annoying symptoms, how to deal with them at work, and how to make strong support networks. We'll talk about the law (yes, you do have rights!) and how to make a policy that supports women going through menopause at work. We'll also talk about how to have tough conversations with bosses and coworkers.

Hold on tight, and get ready to feel strong. We're going to use those hot flashes to make things better, because you deserve to do well at work, menopause and all.

Part 1: Menopause: Understanding the Workplace Impact

Chapter 1: It's Not Just in Your Head: The Science of Menopause Symptoms & Their Effect on Work

Imagine that you are in the middle of giving a very important speech when all of a sudden, a wave of heat hits you. It's so scary that for a moment your mind goes blank and your face turns bright red like a beetroot. Or, imagine that you are trying to negotiate a complicated contract but your brain is so clouded with confusion that you can't remember important details or put together words that make sense. Sense a pattern?
You're not crazy; you're just going through the menopause roller coaster. But here's the thing: knowing the science behind those annoying symptoms is the first thing that will help you deal with them at work and feel comfortable asking for help when you need it.

Hormonal Chaos: The People Who Work Behind the Scenes

Menopause is like a song that has gone wrong. Hormones, mostly estrogen and progesterone, take a break from being the director. What was once a beautiful tune turns into a discordant mess that affects your memory and your ability to control the temperature. These are the main people to blame:

• Nose active estrogen: estrogen does more than just keep your periods regular. Mood, sleep, focus, and even the flexibility of your skin are all affected by it. It costs your body a lot when it comes to its end.

• The Exit of Progesterone: This hormone, which works with estrogen, helps keep mood and sleep in check. Its removal makes the effects of estrogen loss worse.

• Androgens Stay: Yes, women also make male hormones like testosterone. The tricky part is that androgens take over when estrogen and progesterone leave the party. This can cause hair to grow in places you don't want it to and annoying pimples.

Symptoms Other Than the Hot Flash: The Many Other Effects

Women going through menopause often have hot flashes, but that's only the beginning. You'll have a lot of different signs during menopause. Some go away fast, others last a long time, and everyone has a different experience. Here is a list of people who cause trouble at work:

• Temper tantrums: Hot flashes and night sweats are not only uncomfortable, but they can also make it hard to concentrate, give you low energy, and even mess up your looks for important meetings.

• Who Takes Your Sleep: Changes in hormones keep you up at night. Lack of sleep or sleepless nights can make you tired, irritable, and more likely to make mistakes at work.

• Brain Freeze: Forgetting things, having trouble finding words, and having trouble focusing—welcome to the wonderful world of menopause brain fog. You might feel like cotton candy is stuck in your head instead of your usually sharp mind.

• Roller Coaster of Mood: A lot of different emotions, from worry and anger to mild sadness, can happen during menopause. It's harder to deal with stress at work and in relationships when your emotions are all over the place.

• And the rest of them... The list keeps going – Vaginal dryness, joint pain, headaches, and changes in weight are some of the things that every woman goes through during menopause. It needs to be fixed if it's getting in the way of your work.

The Unknown Effects of Work: There's More to It Than Just Being Sick

Symptoms of menopause are more than just annoying. They have effects on your job in the real world:

• Drops in Productivity: Being tired, having brain fog, or being anxious can make it hard to always do your best. There are tight deadlines, poor quality, and a lot of sorrow.

•The Confidence Gap: It's clear when you don't believe in your own skills. It's easy to feel like an imposter, which can stop you from sticking up for yourself or taking risks.

• Sick days and hidden costs: When you miss work because of painful symptoms or doctor's appointments, it affects not only you but also your team and, in the end, the business.

• Presenteeism: the risk of dragging yourself to work when you're sick or not paying attention. You make more mistakes, and your long-term health gets worse.

The good news is that you can lessen these effects by being aware of them, learning how to control yourself, and having a supportive workplace. In this fight, knowledge really is power.

Next, we'll talk about how to deal with those annoying symptoms at work, which will help you get back in control and feel like yourself (or even better!) again at work.

Pay attention to brain fog: what's going on and how it ruins your workday

Think about this: You're talking about a project plan when all of a sudden, the words you use every day seem to go away. Names and numbers get lost, and that great idea you had just now? Oh, gone. It's not just embarrassing; it's scary. What the heck is brain fog during menopause?

•It's real! Brain fog is a real symptom that has been proven by study, even though it sounds vague. It doesn't mean you're less smart or that you're getting dementia early.

•The Link Between Estrogens: Studies show that estrogen is very important for brain function, especially when it comes to memory, attention, and language skills. When your levels go down, your brain doesn't work as well as it used to.

Factors that make things worse: What's with the terrible irony?

Stress (hello, tight deadlines!) and not getting enough sleep (thanks, menopause!) make brain fog worse. It keeps going and going.

From Being Angry to Taking Action: How to Get Rid of Brain Fog at Work

Even though the fight is real, you don't have to give up. Let's get rid of this brain fog right away:

• The Basics Are A Must: For easier thinking, it's important to eat well, work out regularly, and get more sleep (even though that can be hard!).

• Lists will save you: You'll find that lengthy to-do lists, written notes, and phone alarms are your new best friends. Don't trust your mind; put it somewhere else!

• Take it apart: Do big jobs seem too much to handle? Break them up into smaller steps that you can handle. This takes some stress off your mind and keeps you on track.

• Cut down on distractions: To focus better, turn off messages, find a quiet place if you can, and do one thing at a time.

• The "Buffer Zone": If you can, try to plan tasks that require a lot of mental energy for when you're at your best. Then, do tasks that are less mentally demanding in between.

Why communication is important: Transparency and Help

When brain fog hits, which it will, being honest can save face:

• A heads-up to coworkers: Saying something like, "Sorry, I'm having some menopausal brain fog today!" can help avoid misunderstandings and make things less weird.

When you talk to your boss: If brain fog is really getting in the way of your work, you might need to have a private talk with your boss to ask for temporary help or changes.
After taking care of the symptoms, long-term solutions and the treatment talk
Even though self-management skills are very helpful, you should talk to your doctor about other treatment choices as well:

• Hormone Replacement Therapy (HRT): For many women, HRT is a game-changer because it replaces the hormones that are lost and helps with a lot of symptoms, like brain fog. Be sure to talk to your doctor about the risks and rewards.

• Supplements and alternative treatments: There are many choices, from herbal treatments to acupuncture. Talk to a doctor or nurse who specializes in menopause to find out what might work best for you.

Don't forget that you're not fighting this battle by yourself. It's frustrating, but you can get your focus back and shine at work again with some strategies, help, and maybe even more treatment choices.

Chapter 2: When Work Feels Impossible: Productivity, Concentration, and the Hidden Challenges

The menopause can make your job feel like a fight in quicksand some days. You get through the day with the help of caffeine and sheer willpower, but your output goes down. Your thoughts are wandering, tasks are looming large, and your sense of competence that you used to have starts to crumble. It makes you want to hide under your desk. It's frustrating when people are going through things that no one else can see. Let's look behind the scenes at how menopause secretly ruins your job by making you doubt your own skills and making you less productive.

The Point Fiasco: The Random Rebellion in Your Brain

Menopause doesn't just make it hard to focus sometimes; it can make it impossible to do anything at all. Your once-reliable ability to focus on a job seems like a long time ago. Distractions that didn't bother you much before now mess up your whole work. A coworker talking across the room, a tapping pen, or the buzzing of an air conditioner can all get in the way of your concentration.

It's not that you're weak or lazy; it's that your brain is having trouble processing information and staying focused because your estrogen levels are changing. When you add in the general mental fatigue that comes with menopause, you have a recipe for putting things off and wasting time looking at your computer screen. Being Low on Energy: Running on Empty

Remember that happy woman who came to work ready to take on the world? During menopause, she is often replaced by a version of herself who is always tired. Not getting enough sleep, whether because of night sweats or insomnia, makes you feel groggy and uninspired. Then there are those quick hot flashes that make you sweat a lot and then get cold, which throws off your work schedule and drains your energy. Menopause can make you feel generally slow, even if you get a good night's sleep. It's like your internal battery is only half full all the time. Everything is affected by this constant low-level fatigue, which makes it harder to push yourself, pay attention in meetings, or get excited about starting new tasks.

The Cost in Feelings: When there is more stress Mood swings caused by menopause or high worry can make work a dangerous place to be emotionally. Small things that used to cause you stress now cause big feelings that make you upset and unable to calm down. When you're irritable and stress is building, it's hard to work together with other people.

Menopause can make you less strong generally, even if you're not going through major emotional changes. You get tired of juggling your demanding job and your body's unpredictable needs all the time. This makes you more likely to feel stressed and burned out. When imposter syndrome hits, it can make you lose confidence. When you can't concentrate, feel in control of your feelings, or get much done, self-doubt starts to creep in. That inner critic that was only a whisper before gets stronger. You start to question every choice you make because you're afraid that your coworkers will notice when you make a mistake or that your boss will doubt your skills. This anxiety makes you feel even worse about yourself and your performance, which is a vicious loop.

How to Handle the Unseen Work of Menopause

Mental and social problems are hard enough on their own, but menopause adds a whole new level of problems with getting things done at work. The sneaky trips to the bathroom to change clothes that are wet with sweat or deal with periods that come on out of the blue. The never-ending search for a quiet spot to cool off after a hot flash. The trips to the doctor and the store that take time away from work. Even though these jobs don't seem like much, they add up and take away time and mental space from your real job.

The Way Forward: Ways to Get Back into the Swing of Things at Work

This chapter isn't about dwelling on the problems; it's about getting a handle on them so we can start fighting back. Next, we'll talk about how to deal with these secret problems in the real world:

• Productivity Hacks: looking at ways to manage your time, block out noise, and break up jobs into manageable chunks that work with the way your energy changes naturally.

• Techniques for Reducing Stress: learning how to deal with stress at work, calming down when you feel too much, and practicing techniques you can use at work.

• Making yourself stronger: Advice on how to make good habits, sleep better, and improve your emotional skills so that you can handle the stresses of work and menopause better.

When imposter syndrome hits, it can make you lose confidence.

This change is very subtle, and it can eat away at you without you even realizing it. That voice inside you that used to give you a good dose of confidence starts to sprinkle doubt into it. When you go through menopause, your old fears can get worse, making you question every choice you make and see yourself negatively compared to coworkers. This slow loss of confidence can happen to anyone, even women who have always been very sure of themselves.

The way it works at work is like this:
• Analytical Sitting: Every email and report is looked over and over again. You might not be able to do your work well because you're afraid of making a mistake.

• Having doubts about yourself: You start to doubt your efforts and ideas. You're afraid to speak up in meetings, even when you have something important to say.

• Fear of Feedback: Even constructive feedback, which you used to see as a chance to improve, now feels like an attack on your character, which makes you feel even worse about your own shortcomings.

• Giving up on the promotion: When great chances come up, you don't take them because your imposter syndrome tells you, "Someone else is more qualified." You get in the way of your own progress.

• Making Mistakes Bigger: In your thoughts, a small mistake is seen as a huge failure. You don't just move on from it; instead, you think about it and beat yourself up, which makes you feel even worse about your confidence.

This is why imposter syndrome is so bad during menopause

You need to know that this isn't "just in your head." The real causes are in the body and in society:

• Hormone Chaos: Changing estrogen levels can make you feel more anxious and harsh on yourself. Mood swings that come with menopause can make you feel even less sure of yourself.

• The Stage of Life: Many women are rethinking their jobs and future goals around the time they go through menopause. This natural tendency to think about yourself can make you more sensitive to what other people see as flaws.

• The ugly head of ageism: People still treat older women less than they deserve, sometimes in subtle ways and sometimes not so subtly. Even if you are aware that you don't want those messages, they can get into your mind and make you doubt yourself even more.

How to Stop the Confidence Drain: Get Back to Being Your Powerhouse Self

You can get over fake syndrome caused by menopause, but it will take work. Let's get this over with:

• Stand up to the critic: When those bad thoughts come up, you should question them. Are they based on truth or fear? Tell the difference between your menopause mood swings and your real skills.

• Keep your eye on the wins: Making a "wins list" of all the things you've done well is a good idea. Keep going back to it, especially when you start to doubt yourself.

• The Power of Positive comments: Ask a trusted coworker or mentor for positive comments. It can be very reassuring to see your skills through someone else's eyes.

There are times when you need to act sure of yourself even though you don't really feel that way. If you stand up straighter and speak up in meetings, your brain will start to catch up.

• Look for your cheerleaders: People who believe in you and help you will make you stronger. Their help is very important for fighting that sneaky   inner   judge.

Remember that you've been through tough situations before and will get through this one too. Going through menopause doesn't make you less valuable, less experienced, or less likely to be successful at work in the future.

You have the power to turn off imposter syndrome and reconnect with the strong, capable woman you know you are.

Chapter 3: The Emotional Toll: Anxiety, Mood Swings, and Their Impact on Your Work Life

Menopause isn't just changes in your body. It can send you into a storm of feelings that will make you feel like a different person than you normally are. You'll be on top of things one minute and lost in tears in the bathroom of the office the next. This emotional roller coaster can make you angry, embarrassed, and just plain worn out, and it can show up at work in ways you might not even notice at first.

The Danger of Mood Swings: Going from 0 to Overwhelmed in Seconds

Image your feelings as a volume button that breaks all of a sudden. Small irritations that didn't bother me much before now cause big emotions. All in the same morning, I snapped at a coworker over a misunderstanding, got very angry at a traffic jam, and then broke down in tears over a lost file. Unpredictability turns into the new normal for you.

You're not weak or crazy. Neurotransmitters that control mood are greatly affected by changes in estrogen levels. When you add in not getting enough sleep and the general stress of life and work, it's easy to feel like you have no control over your situation.

These changes in how you feel don't just happen when you're not working. They get into every part of your work life and make it harder to stay focused, make friends at work, and give off an air of calm ability that is typical of professionals.

Stress: Your Unwanted New Coworker

Many women experience a rise in anxiety during menopause or find that their anxiety conditions get worse. That familiar feeling of worry could turn into a deep unease that makes even simple jobs feel hard. You can't stop thinking about the worst things that could happen because your mind is racing with "what if" scenarios.

This worry feeds into a loop that makes things worse. You question your choices when you're afraid of being looked at closely. Stage fright before speeches can make you unable to do anything. Some days it's scary just to walk into the office because you're waiting for the next wave of sudden fear.

Depression's Shadow: When Thrills Wear Off

Even though mood changes are more noticeable, the bad moods that can come with menopause are just as annoying. You lose interest in things that used to make you happy, like your job. Instead of your usual excitement, you might feel apathy or cynicism. It gets harder to care and get motivated. Somewhere deep inside you feels guilty that you're not doing your best and are letting your team down.

Workplace Fallout: The Real Effects of Emotional Upheaval

Changes in emotions cause problems in both subtle and not-so-subtle ways:
Relationships at Work Go through: Mood changes make it hard for coworkers to trust you. They might feel like they have to be careful

because they don't know how you'll respond next. Chances thrown away: When you're anxious, you might not be able to speak up in meetings, volunteer for new projects, or network, all of which are good for your job.

The Damage to Reputation: No matter how good your work is, having public emotional meltdowns or reactions that aren't like you hurts your professional image.
Less obvious Health and happiness: Having to deal with strong feelings all the time is very hard. You're more likely to get burned out and cynical, and you don't have as much spare time to handle general work duties.

Now is the time to act: Ways to Keep Your Emotions in Check

You don't have to just accept this mental chaos, which is good news. Now is the time to fight back! Let's look at some ways to deal with these problems:
Food, exercise, and sleep are all basic things that can have a big impact on your happiness. Putting these first helps your general health and emotional strength during menopause.

How to Calm Your Anxious Mind: Learn how to relax with deep breathing, mindfulness, and guided visualization. These skills can help you both before and during anxiety attacks.

The Power of Therapy to Change Things: Cognitive behavioral therapy (CBT) teaches people how to change their negative thought habits, deal with anxiety, and find healthy ways to deal with problems.

When you should see a doctor: Don't be afraid to talk to your doctor if your worry, mood swings, or low moods are making your life very hard. Some medicines, like some drugs or HRT, can help some women. Why disclosure is important: Should You Tell Someone or Not? It can be hard to talk about problems at work. You might want to get help from HR or a trusted mentor to figure out the culture of your company. A private chat with a helpful boss can lead to small changes that really help, like being able to change your meeting times or having a quiet place to work together, etc. Remember that you're not the only one going through this. Having a more open conversation about mental health is good for everyone.

How to Calm Your Anxious Mind: Useful Tools for Stress Relief at Work

No matter where you are, anxiety can happen. But the stresses of the job make it even harder to handle. When you start to feel panicked, you need quick, quiet, and effective ways to deal with it in a business setting. Let's make a toolkit for dealing with worry at work:

Getting a sense of grounding through: When your mind is running, use your senses to bring yourself back to the present. Pay close attention to five things you can see, four things you can feel, three things you can hear, two things you can smell, and one thing you can taste. How Breath Works: Your body will relax when you breathe deeply into your belly. Slowly breathe in for four counts, hold for four counts, and then slowly breathe out for four counts. Do it several times. If you can, find a quiet place to do this. This is fine to do at your work, though.

Break for mini-visualization: Close your eyes and picture a peaceful place, like a beach, a forest, or any other place that makes you feel calm. Pay attention to the details and use all of your senses. This short break can help your nervous system get back to normal.

Progressive Muscle Relaxation: Tense and relax groups of muscles all over your body in a quiet way, starting at your toes and working your way up. This helps ease the tension in your body, which is often linked to worry.

How the Water Works: A quick splash of cold water on your face or arms can help you stop feeling hopeless. Please excuse yourself to use the bathroom for a moment to do this easy reset. Building a foundation for emotional resilience outside of work hours

Those techniques aren't the only way to deal with worry. In addition, it's about making you stronger overall:

Meditation and being mindful: If you practice for just 10 minutes every day, your brain will learn to handle worried thoughts better. You can get great guided apps to help you get started.

Talk It Out: Therapy gives you a safe place to look into what's causing your worry, come up with ways to deal with it, and learn how to change negative thought patterns.

Physical Release: Working out is a natural way to relieve stress. Find something you enjoy doing, like dancing, brisk walks, or yoga, and make it a steady part of your life.

The Sleep Connection: Not getting enough sleep on a regular basis makes worry worse. For mental health, especially during menopause, putting good sleep hygiene first is very important.

How to Use "No" to Your Advantage: Sometimes it's important to lighten your load. Saying "no" to unimportant responsibilities at work and in your personal life will give you more time to take care of yourself and   relax.

It's a sign of power, not weakness, to ask for help. If your anxiety is making your life very hard, don't be afraid to talk to your doctor or a mental health expert. There are solutions that work, and you don't have to go through this alone.

Part 2: Strategies for Success at Work

Chapter 4: Building Your Menopause Work Toolkit: Practical Solutions for Symptom Management on the Job

Think about this: you're about to go to a big meeting when you feel a familiar wave of heat coming up your neck. Or maybe the feared brain fog hits while you're working on something hard. The signs of menopause tend to show up at the worst times, making it hard to get work done. It doesn't need to be this way, though. Now is the time to take charge and put together your own personalized menopause work toolkit. This will be a collection of strategies and resources that will help you handle the expected flare-ups with grace and lessen their negative effects.

How to Control Hot Flashes at Work: Your Plan for Cooling Down Women going through menopause often have hot flashes, but they don't have to hold you hostage at work. By using more than one method, you can lessen their strength, shorten their length, and hide their effects:

• The Dress Code Conundrum: If your job lets you, wear natural fabrics that let air flow, like cotton or linen. Layers are your best friend. A cardigan or coat that you can easily put on and take off gives you options when your body temperature changes.

• The Arsenal at Your Desk: A small fan for yourself can save your life. Pick a model that is quiet, doesn't stand out, and cools specific areas. On the go, a cold-water bottle or a spray that cools your face and arms can help you feel better quickly.

• Changes to your environment: If you can, move away from heat sources like heaters or sunny windows. If you can, ask to switch desks or leave a window open.

• Be aware of triggers: Write down the things that cause your hot flashes, like caffeine, spicy foods, and worry. Some things can't be helped, but limiting the ones you can makes a difference.

• The Power of Deep Breathing: Taking slow, steady breaths can help calm the nervous system and even make hot flashes less intense. Learn this method when you're feeling calm so you can use it quickly when you need to.

Getting rid of brain fog: getting your focus back

The fog of menopause can make you lose the focus you used to take for granted. This can be frustrating, and you may worry that you'll lose your professional edge. Even though you can't get rid of brain fog totally, these tips will help you think more clearly during those important work moments:

• How to Trick Your Brain: If fog comes in, keep things simple. Split big jobs into small steps and work on one thing at a time. Externalize your memories by using lots of notes, alarms, and calendar alerts. Don't put too much stress on your memory.

• Strategic Timing: Figure out when you work best on mentally demanding tasks and plan them for that time. Keep that focused time safe and limit interruptions as much as possible.

• Talking Low-Key: If you suddenly get brain fog, don't be afraid to buy some time. Saying "Let me think about that and get back to you" is better than giving a wrong answer.

Keep yourself hydrated: Even slight dehydration makes it harder to think clearly. Keep a water bottle by your desk and drink from it often all day.

• Keeping your brain healthy: a well-balanced diet full of whole foods helps your brain work well. Keep healthy food like fruit or nuts on hand to avoid low blood sugar that makes it harder to concentrate.

Going Beyond the Surface: Getting to the Causes

Strategies for the present time are very important, but don't forget the power of long-term solutions:

• Talk about The Doctor: Talk to your doctor about treatment choices like Hormone Replacement Therapy (HRT), which helps many women a lot with not only hot flashes but also brain fog and other cognitive problems.

• Sleep as a Superpower: It's important to make good sleep habits a priority. Better sleep helps you focus at work. You can do this by sticking to a regular bedtime routine or by looking at your sleep surroundings.

• Taking care of your stress that way: Every sign of menopause gets worse with long-term stress. Make time for ways to relax, even if it's just for a short time during the job. Also, exercise is a great way to relieve stress.

Remember that this is a constant process of getting better. Try these tactics out, keep track of what works, and over time, make your toolkit better. Even though menopause can be rough at times, you can handle it and keep up your working pace if you prepare well.

How to Deal with the Unexpected: Periods and Bladder Problems The menopause changes both how often you have periods and how well you can control your body. Periods can change quickly, get heavier, or come closer together, which can catch you off guard. Weak pelvic floor muscles, on the other hand, can cause embarrassing or necessary leaks, especially when sneezing, laughing, or being stressed at work. Don't let these problems rule you; planning ahead is the only way to win.

• Your emergency kit for your period: Put together a covert pouch with the things you need: extra-absorbent pads or tampons for days when you don't expect to be having a lot of leaks, a spare pair of underwear, and discreet feminine wipes. For peace of mind, keep this in your desk box or work bag.

• Keeping you dry and boosting your confidence: pantyliners are your new secret tool. To keep them fresh, change them often. To add an extra measure of safety, discreet bladder control pads that look like regular maxi pads can be used.

• Mapping the Facilities: Know the fastest way to get to the bathroom and try to find single-stall bathrooms that aren't too busy so you can handle things without feeling rushed or self-conscious.

• Changes to your hydration and timing: It's important to stay hydrated, but don't drink a lot of water all at once. Take it easy during the day and remember to take breaks to go to the bathroom before important events or meetings.

• Why pelvic floor exercises are so important: Kegel movements make the muscles that help you control your bladder stronger.

You can look online for simple routines you can do at your desk.

They're private (no one will know you're doing them!) and very helpful over time.

The Problem of Vaginal Dryness: Discomfort and Tough Conversations

During menopause, vaginal dryness becomes more common. This can cause pain, itching, and less natural moisture. This can make sitting at work for long amounts of time very uncomfortable and may even make it harder to concentrate and keep your mood up. Here's what you need to do:

• Relief at your desk: Small, water-based oils can help for a short time. Search for small ones that fit in your bag. Stay away from items that are based on petroleum jelly for this area.

• Clothes That Matter: If you want to avoid itching during the day, wear soft, breathable underwear and pants that don't fit too tightly.

• Beyond Lubricants: Vaginal moisturizers work better and last longer than lubricants. Talk to your doctor or pharmacist about over-the-counter choices. If over-the-counter options don't work, you may want to look into prescription treatments.

• When having sex hurts: Women who are still sexually active may find that vaginal dryness makes sex painful or uncomfortable.

Don't suffer alone; you need to have an honest talk with your doctor. Lubricants, longer foreplay, and maybe even estrogen products that you put on your skin can help.

The Big Talks: Doctors and Partners

These are touchy subjects, but it's important to talk about them openly. Having these talks with your partner is a good idea if they are affecting your health. It can feel unsafe to talk about dryness and changing sexual needs. Pick a calm time and frame it from your point of view. Think about your own experience and work together to find understanding and answers.

• Your doctor or nurse: Make it clear what kind of pain or trouble dryness causes. Don't let being ashamed stop you from getting help. You can get care in a lot of different ways, and your doctor will help you find the best one for you.

Don't forget that you're not the only one going through this. Get useful tools for solving problems and don't be afraid to ask for help when you need it. Dealing with these problems head-on gives you the power to regain your happiness and well-being at work and elsewhere.

Chapter 5: Cooling Down (Literally & Figuratively): Temperature Control, Dress Codes, and Managing Hot Flashes

Imagine that you are giving a talk when it happens: your body gets really hot, your skin turns beetroot red, and sweat starts to form on your forehead. All eyes are on you, and you want an exit hatch more than anything. Hot flashes are more than just a physical pain; they can also cause stress at work and hurt the professional image you've worked hard to build. On the other hand, a flash of heat doesn't always mean a wreck.

You can win those temperature fights with proactive strategies, smart adaptation, and maybe even a reevaluation of the norms at work.

When Your Ideal Temperature Is The Arctic Blast of Everyone Else The temperature in the office is rarely a neutral subject, but for women going through menopause, it can be a danger. The people you work with are wearing sweaters, but you want to take off your clothes. It can be annoying and even embarrassing when your hot flashes make your problem clear in a way that no one else can understand. Leave the hopelessness behind and get to work:

Know what your rights are: Find out if your job or area has rules about the temperature ranges that are allowed in offices. The best way to fight for yourself is to know what you're talking about.

The Solutions for One: Changes in the temperature of the whole building may not be possible, but focus on what you can change. It can really help to have a strong work fan, a cooling spray, or an ice pack tucked away in your clothes.

Setting up a strategy: Environmental heat factors can be kept to a minimum by asking for a desk that isn't in full sunlight, next to a hot radiator, or in a stuffy corner. It helps to make even small changes.

What Really Happened: A nice one-on-one with your office boss might help you figure things out. Without giving away too many personal details, talk about how the setting affects your work and suggest ways to make things better, such as having a fan at your desk or being able to take short "cooling-off" breaks.

The Dress Code Challenge: Being Professional vs. Being Useful As women go through menopause, strict dress rules become their worst enemy. Blazers make it hard to breathe, itchy fabrics make hot flashes worse, and not being able to change your clothes makes you even more frustrated. Your rebellious side wants to wear a tank top and shorts, but in reality, you need to find a middle ground that works for you:

Fabric is All That: Instead of synthetics, choose natural fibers that let air flow, like cotton, linen, or light wools. Wearing sports clothes that wick away sweat while looking like smart casual clothes could save your life.

Use the Power of Layers: You need to have a sweater, scarf, or light jacket that you can easily take off during hot flashes and put back on when you start to feel cold again.

The Color Conundrum: Light colors keep you cool, but they also make sweat spots stand out more. In places where you can see sweat, choose darker colors on purpose.

Freedom of Footwear: Choose shoes that let air flow through them whenever you can, or keep a "desk pair" of sandals on hand for when you're having a hot flash and your feet want to get out of those stuffy boots.

To advocate is to act: Start a private conversation with HR about easing up on the dress rule during months with bad weather. For a large part of their staff, menopause is not a trend but a fact of life.

Taking care of the mortification: When Hot Flashes Get Out in Public

Everyone has had that bright red flush, the sweat that you can see, and the stuttering phrase in the middle of a meeting. Hot flashes can happen at any time. You can't completely stop them, but you can choose how you react:

The Defense of Humor: "Menopause moment, bear with me!" can help ease the stress and, surprisingly often, get other women who are going through the same thing to nod their heads in agreement.

It's a temporary guarantee: As you and those around you feel stressed, tell yourself, "This will pass quickly." It makes things less awkward and gives you a chance to regroup.

The Technique for Distraction: Keep a cold-water bottle nearby, take a step back and splash cool water on your face, or use a cooling wipe without drawing attention to yourself. The act of slowing down also makes you feel better.

Power-Up After Flash: If you can, take a moment to get back together alone. Take a few deep breaths and give yourself a pep talk in the mirror to calm down before getting back into the fight.

The Hidden Cost: How Hot Flashes Get in the Way of Your Work Hot flashes have effects that go beyond being uncomfortable and embarrassed for a short time. They make you less confident and less happy at work over time:

Work Efficiency Go down: Interruptions to cool down, change sweaty clothes, or clear your mind after a flash eat away at time and focus that could be used for work.

The Loss of Confidence: You might not speak up in meetings or take on public roles because you're afraid of looking red at an important time. This can slow your professional growth.

Adding to your anxiety: The fact that your hot flashes can happen at any time adds to your stress and fear, making you feel less in control and lowering your mood even on "cooler" days.

Putting out the candle: It takes a lot of mental and physical energy to deal with the constant changes in temperature and discomfort. This wears you out for both work and home life.

How People See Things: Fighting Stigma and Changing the Conversation

It's easy to believe the society messages that tell us menopause makes us weak or that we have to put up a stiff upper lip during hot flashes. It's time to change that story:

Don't blame yourself for your body; Remember that hot flashes are a normal part of your body and not a sign of a bad personality. You're not becoming less skilled; your body is just getting used to it.

Being Kind to Yourself as a Strength: Criticizing yourself for the fight only makes you feel worse about yourself. Take care of yourself with kindness, just like you would a sick coworker.

The Effects of Silence That Spread: You keep up the stereotype every time you hide a hot flash or say you're "hormonal," Simply say that you need a fan or a short break to cool down to make the talk more normal.

To Know is to Have Power: Learn everything you can about menopause. Knowing the science behind the signs gives you the power to make smart decisions and speak up for yourself and others.

How Advocacy Works: Changing the way things are done at work You deserve to work in a place that understands and supports the facts of menopause. Big changes usually take time, but here's how to speed things up:

Find your friends: Find other women at work who probably understand your problems and do it in a quiet way. Make a network of people who can help you, share tips, and come up with answers.

Outside of the Bathroom Not loudly: In the workplace, hold a relaxed lunch-and-learn about menopause. Think about how it affects production and the health of your employees as well as the health of women.

Set a good example: Make it normal to take small breaks or keep a fan at your desk to cool down. Showing others that taking care of your symptoms is an important part of self-care will push them to do the same.

A proposal for policy: Work with an understanding HR person to talk about possible changes to the dress code, more flexible break options, or even menopause education materials for managers and employees.

Remember that fighting for change isn't just about you. You're making the world a better place to work by recognizing that people have different needs at different times of their lives. That's a powerful memory to leave behind!

Chapter 6: Brain Fog Be Gone: Tips for Focus, Memory, and Mental Clarity

Menopause can make you forget where you put your car keys, can't remember the name of that important client, or feel like your brain has turned into fuzzy cotton wool. It takes a lot of work to do things that used to feel easy. The good news is that even though menopause does make it harder to think clearly, you can fight back with strategies that will help you get your thoughts back on track and make brain fog less of a problem at work.

Menopause makes you forget things, which is called "understanding the enemy."

Brain fog is not a medical condition; it's just a word that women use to describe times when they forget things, have trouble focusing, and feel mentally scattered. It's important to know that you're not crazy and that you're not the only one going through this. Here are the main people to blame:

• Estrogen's Retreat: Estrogen is a very important hormone for brain function, especially when it comes to memory, attention, and speaking clearly. Your neurons aren't firing as smoothly as they used to because its amounts are going down.

• Not getting enough sleep: If you have hot flashes, night sweats, or trouble sleeping, your brain can't get the restful sleep it needs to focus and remember things. It's a vicious loop because not getting enough sleep makes brain fog worse.

• Too much stress: During menopause, people often have to deal with extra stress from things like kids moving out, parents getting older, or job changes. Cortisol is a hormone that makes it harder to think clearly and is released when you are under a lot of stress.

• Disruptive Role of Mood Swings: The anxiety and mood swings that come with menopause can take your mind off of things, making it even harder to think straight.

The War in the Workplace: How brain fog gets in the way of your work

Brain fog doesn't just make it hard to find your keys; it really messes up your workday:

• The Productivity Plunge: Small jobs seem huge, choices seem too hard, and putting things off becomes your new best friend. Not meeting goals and having a long list of things to do add to the stress.

• More mistakes: typos, oversights, and math mistakes happen more often, making you do more work and losing faith in your own skills.

• Communication Breakdown: Having trouble remembering words makes talks awkward, which makes you angry and worries that you sound less articulate than before.

• The Memory Loss of Small Details: Names, times, and other details that used to be easy to remember now fade away when you need them, making you feel awkward and anxious in client meetings or team discussions.

Brain Fog on the Job: How to Beat the Battle Plan

Getting your focus back doesn't mean finding a magic bullet. Instead, it means putting together a full set of strategies. In the same way that target practice makes you better at something, this will test your skills every day. Okay, the important thing is to be consistent and kind to yourself:

• The Important Things Matter: As much as possible, put sleep first, even if that means making a strict bedtime plan or talking to your doctor about how to deal with symptoms at night. To keep your blood sugar level, eat regularly, drink plenty of water, and make time for short bursts of activity every day.

• Turn off your brain: Don't put more stress on your memory, which is already bad. A detailed to-do list, phone alarms, and calendar notes can help you stay on track.

• Break It Up: Being too busy is bad for you. Split big jobs into small, manageable steps and take a break between each one to clear your mind.

• One task at a time saves the day: Close browser tabs that aren't needed and turn off phone notifications. Focus on the job at hand, even if it's a little fuzzy, to avoid making mistakes.

• Accept the "Do Not Disturb" message: Set aside chunks of time to focus on difficult jobs when you can. Calls can be directed to someone else, the door shut, and a nice "Unavailable for an hour" sign.

The Power of Strategic Environment and Timing

You can't stop brain fog from happening, but you can get the most out of your clear thinking by choosing when and where to do those mentally difficult tasks:

• Figure out your busiest time: Notice when your mind is at its sharpest, even if it's only for a short time. Protect that time very carefully for the work that you find hardest, and try to avoid meetings and other interruptions as much as possible during that time.

• The environment is very important: Find a quiet place when your brain fog is bad. Noise-canceling headphones, a place with no other things going on, or even working outside can help you concentrate again.

• Problem-solving ahead of time: Plan for possible problems. Writing down important points you want to make before a long meeting is helpful. You could also make a short tip sheet with names and information you might need.

"I'll Get Back to You" Mantra: Don't worry if your mind goes blank right now. Spend your money on time instead. "That's a great question, let me check on that and circle back" or even "Interesting point, let me do a deeper dive into that for you" save your life.

Hacks for Mental Agility: How to Get Your Brain to Focus

There are times when you need a few tricks to get your brain working again. Here is your set of tools:

• The Sensory Jolt: A short change in excitement can help you get back on track. Get some fresh air by going outside, splashing cold water on your face, or sucking on a strong mint.

• Boost Your Body Movement: If you can, do some jumping jacks or pushups at your desk. If not, go for a quick walk around the block. When your blood flow goes up, your brain wakes up.

• The Word Retrieval Workout: Play word association games when you can't remember that important word. You could think of similar words or ideas, or you could even picture the thing. It often helps you remember things.

• Turning Focus into a Game: Time yourself for 25 minutes and push yourself to work hard on one job for that long. It is possible to work in short, focused bursts even when your brain is foggy.

The Honest Conversation: When to Tell Someone, You Have Brain Fog
It's hard to decide if you should talk to your boss or coworkers about your brain fog. There are good and bad points:

• Possible Advantages: Being honest can help people understand and take away the worry of hiding your problems. You might be able to change dates or have team members be more flexible when you're having a rough patch.

• The Risk Factor: Bias is a real problem. Pick carefully who you tell, and base it on your desire to do your best work while making some possible adjustments.

• The Partial-Disclosure Option: If going all the way feels risky, say something like, "I haven't been sleeping well. Could we talk about this again tomorrow?" or "I need a quick walk to clear my head. I'll be right back."

Remember that brain fog is a real condition that can lead to real problems. Even though it's annoying, it doesn't make you less smart or capable. You can handle mental storms and keep your professional edge if you know yourself, use techniques, and look into possible workplace accommodations.

Part 3: Communication & Building Support

Chapter 7: Finding Your Voice at Work: Talking about Menopause without Shame

The quiet that comes with menopause is worse for many women than any hot flash. You deal with your symptoms in private, hiding the sweat spots and saying sorry for "hormonal" moments. You fear the day when your well-built facade falls apart in a very public meltdown. Shame leads to secrecy, and shame leads to being alone. But there is another way. You can let go of the stigma you've put on yourself and choose open conversation. This will lead to a more understanding and welcoming workplace for everyone.

If you hide your problems, you will have to pay a price.

Even though silence seems like the safest choice, it has hidden costs for your job and your own health:

• The Isolation Trap: When you're going through hard times by yourself, you think you're the only one. This makes the fight feel worse and makes you think you're "broken" in some way.

• Misplaced Blame: If you don't talk about your problems, it's easy to see problems at work as personal mistakes, which can hurt your confidence, when the real problem is that you aren't treating your symptoms, which is holding you back.

• Chances to get help that were missed: Your boss or a coworker who "gets it" might be able to make changes or give you easy tips that make all the difference. The doors close when it's quiet.

• Stigma that won't go away: If you don't talk about menopause, it supports the idea that it's embarrassing and something you should deal with without showing any emotion. You don't change that story when you have the chance to.

You have the power to choose: levels of disclosure

When you talk about menopause, you don't have to shout about your hot flashes. You have the right to be alone. It comes down to picking the amount of honesty that works for you and fits with the way things are done at work:

• The Trusted Confidant: Start small by telling one helpful coworker, an HR person, or a mentor outside of work. Having someone to talk to makes things easier.

• The Need-to-Know Explanation: Tell your boss, "I'm having hot flashes and trouble focusing because of a temporary health issue." Can we come up with some changes?" There's no need to say "menopause" out loud unless you want to.

• Advocacy with Anonymity: Can you offer a menopause seminar at work without being seen or give your HR team an informative article in a sneaky way? You can bring about change without talking about your own problems.

• Setting a good example: Say something like, "I need a quick break from my hot flashes!" or "Today I really have brain fog, please bear with me." Others might do what you do to break the ice without giving too much information.

How to Find the Words: Putting together your conversation starters

It can be scary to start these kinds of talks. If you want to be honest while still being professional, here are some techniques you can use:

• With a sympathetic coworker: "You seem like someone who gets it. Are these hot flashes from hell or is it just me?"

• Telling your boss, "I want to take charge of how I handle a temporary health problem." It's making it hard for me to concentrate. Could we talk about making some short-term changes?"

• Making it normal, not too public: "Perimenopause is really bothering me today; does anyone else ever get brain fog like this?"

Looking Forward to the Reactions: From Eye Supports to Side Eyes

Regrettably, not everyone will understand. Get ready for:

• The Uncomfortable Silence: Don't let it stop you. Follow-up, "It affects a lot of women our age, we need to break the taboo to get the support we need."

• The Putting Down Comment: Use facts to back up your claim:

"Menopause affects X% of the workforce." It hurts morale and output to act like it doesn't exist.

• The Unexpected Friend: You never know who will step up—a male coworker whose wife had serious symptoms or a younger woman eager to make the workplace more welcoming in the future.

The Long Game: Keeping the Lines of Communication Open It's not a one-time thing to talk about menopause. It's an ongoing talk as your symptoms change and you figure out what changes to make at work that help the most:

• Check-ins in Place of Whining: Set up regular, short meetings with your boss (if you've told them). Attempt to find answers: "The fan has been amazing, but might it be okay to work remotely on Fridays when my symptoms are worst?"

• How to Do a Heads-Up: In case of brain fog, a polite "I'm a bit fuzzy today, may I follow up in writing to confirm details?" responsibility, not lack of skill.

• Moving forward: Don't say sorry for what you can't do; instead, think about what changes would help you do better. This changes the subject to working together in a good way.

• Boundaries are important: you have the right to privacy. When people ask about your health, a polite but firm "I'm working with my doctor on managing this, thanks for your understanding" will stop them in their tracks.

How to Handle Pushback and Insensitivity When Frustration Flares

Even if you talk to them carefully, they might not listen or say things that are hurtful or not helpful. To stay calm and professional, write your answers ahead of time:

• The "Just Push Through" Attitude: Say something like, "Ignoring this hurts productivity and makes mistakes more likely for everyone." We don't want that to happen.

• Wrong Place for Humor: The awkwardness is now on the ignorant person, who says, "Let's save that joke for when you go through this yourself."

• Data is Your Defense: Make a list of data about how common menopause is in the work force and how much it might cost your company in lost time and employees leaving. Having this makes it harder to brush off your worries.

• Find your friends: When you're being pushed back, people who understand your struggles can help you a lot in fighting for your needs and a larger shift in society.

Besides Yourself: Changes to the system begin with you.

Not only does your voice affect your own experience, it could also change your whole workplace for the better:

• The Ripple Effect: You make it easier for the next woman when you make a menopause problem seem normal or when you stand up to someone who doesn't take it seriously. Just think of it as giving back.

• Information is power. Could you set up a lunch-and-learn on menopause with a women's health expert? Give your HR team some helpful links or even offer to write an anonymous piece for the company newsletter.

• Mentorship Is Important: Is there a younger female coworker you could help? Sharing your stories and the tactics you've come up with gives the next generation strength.

• Policy Push: Work with sympathetic HR reps or coworkers who feel the same way to look into options for a more flexible dress code, ways to control body temperature, or even menopause-specific support groups and tools.

Remember that it only takes one brave person to speak out for systemic change to begin. You become a force for positive change when you speak up for yourself, break down your own internalized shame, and fight against old ways of thinking. It won't always be easy, but hot flashes and foggy brain days will not be the only ones affected.

Chapter 8: Talking to Your Manager: Navigating Difficult Conversations

Discussing hot flashes, brain fog, and feelings that could change quickly with your boss can cause a lot of stress. Being ready, focusing on results, and realizing that you have a lot more power over the course of this conversation than you think are the most important things here.

Prior to the Talk: The Phase of Mindset Shift and Planning

This talk isn't an attempt to get you to feel better; it's a business offer based on your continued contributions to the team:

• Know Your Why: Do you want to be able to change your schedule? A fan for your desk? Just wanting to know what those "off" days are for? Your ask is guided by a clear sense of purpose.

• Don't go into too much depth; you don't have to list every symptom. Pay attention to the ones that have the most effect on your work: "The temperature fluctuations make it difficult to concentrate."

• Approach Focused on Solutions: Before you start making changes, ask yourself things like, "Could I work from home on my hardest days?" or "Could I take a short walk break when I feel overwhelmed?"

• Changing how the story is told: This isn't a weakness; it's just a short-term health problem. Like an employee dealing with migraines, you're constantly looking for ways to reduce the impact of work.

• The Right Time: Do not sneak up on your boss in the hallway. For a focused conversation, ask for a private meeting, even if it's only for 15 minutes.

Getting Around the Details: How to Say It and What to Say

It's very important to find the right words. Let's talk about your choices in a way that fits your relationship with your boss and your comfort level:

• The Low-Key Disclosure: "I'm having trouble focusing because of a short-term health problem." I'd like to talk about changes that will help me stay on track. (Leaves room for interpretation)

• Specific to a symptom: It is hard to focus at work because the temperature changes all the time. Could we look into choices for a desk fan, flexible scheduling, or temperature control?"

• The Strike Before It Happens: (Use if you have a lot of brain fog) "There are times when I get tense or forget things." Please bear with me while I take the necessary steps to handle this.

The data-driven approach: "I'm not the only one who feels this way. A huge portion of the workforce is affected by menopause, and research has shown that workplaces that are supportive have higher output and retention.

Expect and Get Past: Common Concerns and Objections

Plan for less-than-ideal responses and have your counterarguments ready:

• "This is Too Personal" : "I know you don't want to do this, but it affects my work." It's the same as any minor health problem that needs to be accommodated.

• "We Can't Make Exceptions": "I'm not asking for special treatment; I'm just asking for the kind of flexibility that many workplaces offer." Can we look into choices that are fair and doable for everyone?"

• "I Don't Understand": (often with younger bosses or men) "There are great places to learn about menopause and work." I'd be happy to give you some; helping people understand each other is good for everyone.

After the First Ask: Keeping the Conversation Going

Most likely, this won't be the last time we talk about this. Key is constant, open communication:

• The follow-up: "Thank you for being willing to hear this." The change is making things better. We'll check back in a few weeks to see if any changes need to be made.

• Problems with framing: Some days with symptoms are bad. "Today's a rough one, but I'm utilizing the strategies we discussed, and I'll catch up tomorrow." Makes you responsible.

• Speaking out for others: If the talk goes well, suggest that it go on: "Would HR be okay with a short seminar about menopause at work?" That's a problem we all need to solve.

Know what your rights are: When to Take the Talk to the Next Level

It's too bad that not all bosses are open. Don't give up if you are being fired, treated unfairly, or don't feel supported at all:

• Write down everything: Keep track of the things you ask for, how they answer, and the times when your work suffered because of menopause symptoms that weren't dealt with.

• HR as a Friend: Learn about any policies at work that cover health problems or making accommodations for people with disabilities. Get help from HR, especially if you think discrimination is happening.

• How the Power of Group Voice Works: Are there likely to be other women at work who are having the same problems? It can be more important to have a private talk about how to handle HR together.

When Things Get Really Rude: Dealing with Insensitive or Uninformed Bosses

Some bosses will react in ways that will make you want to hide under your desk or cry angry tears, even if you've planned ahead. When things get weird, annoying, or even hurtful, do these things:

People who don't know what to say: "Everyone gets a little fuzzy sometimes" or "My wife just got through it." Answer quietly with facts: "This is way beyond normal tiredness." Managing menopause symptoms in a way that works has been shown to help both me and the company.

• The Inappropriate Joke: When humor is used to avoid feeling bad, it often hides feeling bad. If you say, "It would help me more if we focused on how to minimize work interruptions," you can end the conversation without making things worse.

• The Flat-Out Refusal: "We can't help with every personal issue." This is almost unfair. Tell them in a calm voice, "Menopause isn't a choice; it's biology." A lot of big companies know how important it is to help their employees through this.

Superpowers for Self-Advocacy: Getting Strong Even When It's Tough

These talks can make you feel less sure of yourself. Don't forget:
• It's okay to feel things, but strategy wins: It's okay to feel upset or even angry. Tell a trusted friend about your problems outside of work, and then calm down. Please pay attention to those planned answers.

• You're not begging; you're just asking for fair changes, like someone who is temporarily sick or hurt. The company values your health and how well you do your job.

• Little wins are important: Any progress is good, even if you don't get everything you want. Having a fan at your desk and a plan that is a little less rigid can help you get requests in the future.

• Record, Record, Record: Write down what you talked about, what changes were agreed upon, and any times when a lack of help directly affected your work. In the long run, this will protect you.

The Red Flag Zone: When the Air Quality at Work Is Too Bad

Unfortunately, your health and happiness will never be a priority at some places of work because they are so stuck in the past. When you need to take a stronger stance:

• Your mental health is bad: You are more stressed out about having this talk than you are about the symptoms themselves. That can't go on forever.

• Changes to performance reviews: All of a sudden, you're getting bad reviews about your menopause symptoms, even though you've tried to be open and honest.

• Isolation and shame: The setting makes you feel embarrassed or ashamed to even bring up the subject, which hurts your sense of belonging.

The Next Level: HR, lawyer choices, and Knowing How Much You're Worth

If the good intentions you put in are met with anger or negative consequences, it's time to make more serious moves:

• HR as a Lifeline (or Not): Be careful when you talk to HR. In an ideal world, they'd be on your side to make sure fairness and respect. But unfortunately, some HR teams have the same old-fashioned views as managers.

• The Power of Law: Find out if your company, state, or country has any rights against discrimination or disability caused by menopause. This information gives you power.

• Get help from someone else: You might not know about some of your choices until you talk to a reliable employment lawyer or a group that fights for women's rights at work during menopause.

• Know how much you're worth: Is this job worth the damage it does to your mental and physical health in the worst case? Walking away and finding a new job where everyone is valued is sometimes the bravest thing you can do.

Remember that you're not going through this alone. It takes guts to speak up for yourself, even when it's hard. That's why we're working to change the conversation and make workplaces more welcoming by design. You might not win every fight, but you're building a world where no woman has to suffer in silence or give up her job because of menopause.

Chapter 9: The Power of Peer Support: Finding Allies and Building Community at Work

The quiet that comes with menopause can make you feel like you're fighting an enemy you can't see by yourself. But the truth is that if you look around your workplace, you'll probably see other women who are also fighting the same battles against hot flashes, mood swings, and brain fog. Finding those friends and building a community of support can turn your workday from a slew of embarrassing moments into a place where people understand, give useful advice, and even share some much-needed humor.

How to Find Your Tribe: Trying to Find Possible Allies

Some people might not be open, but you might be shocked at who comes through as a source of support:

• The Likely Suspects: your main targets are middle-aged women. Don't forget about younger women, though; they could become allies in the future or have helped mums or partners through menopause.

• More than just age or gender: Allies come in many forms, such as a male coworker whose wife had symptoms that made her very sick or someone who wants to promote acceptance.

• Watch and interact: Take note of who rolls their eyes when meetings are held in places that are too warm or who seems to be okay with having a "fuzzy brain" moment. "This menopause heat isn't a joke, right?" is a good way to start a talk.

• The Pros of Shopping Online: You can connect with others who may be going through the same problems in a private way through business intranets, women's groups, or even industry-specific social media.

Making a Safe Space: From Small Talk to a Helpful Community

Building a real peer support network is more than just letting off steam in the break room. Here's how to make everyone feel like they fit and give each other power:

• Start small. Starting a group can be scary, but having a coffee chat with one person is easier. Don't talk too much about your health; instead, talk about shared situations.

• Humor as a Healer: Being able to laugh together about things like forgetting words or having sudden sweat attacks takes away the shame and brings people together.

• Sharing useful tips: what helps someone with brain fog could save your life. Set up a casual tip swap to stop feeling like you're floundering alone.

• Making the Talk More Normal: It's not a bad thing to bring up menopause in a team setting; for example, "Brain fog is setting in. Can we talk about this again tomorrow?"

• There is strength in numbers: Talking to management or HR about bigger problems is easier when you have shared information and support.

When Support from Peers Turns into Advocacy: Making Your Voices Hearable

A real support network does more than just listen and offer words of comfort; it also leads to changes at work. Think about whether you can all work together to support things like

• The Lunch & Learn Option: Could you suggest a casual talk about menopause at lunchtime given by a doctor or women's health expert? People are more likely to support it if you frame it around productivity and staff well-being.

• Menopause in the Newsletter: Could you suggest a menopause-themed story for the workplace newsletter? It could be a larger piece about dealing with common health issues at work.

• Mentorship Is Important: Could workers who have been through menopause help those who are just starting to deal with these problems in a more casual way? Sharing knowledge gives everyone more power.

The Ripple Effect says that when you make a visible group of support at work, it affects people outside of work. When managers, HR reps, and coworkers see your network, they will start to question what they thought they knew.

Problems and warnings: Getting to Know Your Workplace Culture

Building a friend support network takes some smarts, especially in workplaces that aren't very forward-thinking:

• Choice Is Important: Being honest is important, but start with people you trust. Choose your confidantes carefully because gossip can get in the way of your goals.

• It's not a party of sadness: Not just complaining, but also on the good things and ways to fix things. This gets support, not ridicule.
• Be open to everyone: Don't make a "menopause club" for only women. Invite allies of all genders, ages, and backgrounds to join the bigger talk.

• Make sure you have limits: When you have a hot flash, you're not a doctor. You can decide how much emotional help you want to give to coworkers.

Taking care of the network: from connecting to building strength as a whole

Making a group of peers to help each other is just the beginning. To get the most out of it, both for yourself and for the rest of the workplace, you need to keep working at it and use some strategy:

• Regularity with Flexibility: Can you set up a "Menopause Monday" coffee break that isn't too formal? Keep it low-key and free so that people can join and leave as they please without feeling pushed.

• The shared set of tools: Everyone can add tips, resources, and even funny memes to a shared document (like a Google Doc or a secure app).

This makes information easy to find and creates a real sense of community.

• Switching roles: Don't make one person the "leader" of everything. One person brings snacks one week, and someone else offers a good article to talk about the next. This kind of shared ownership makes people more committed.

• The Celebration of Wins: Was it possible for someone to work out an open schedule? Have a party! Sharing wins keeps everyone in the group motivated and gives others useful "how to" guides.

How to Use Your Voice for Strategic Advocacy

If you have a strong peer support group, you can use it to push for bigger changes at work that will help everyone:

• Collecting Information: A private, anonymous study at work about how menopause symptoms affect work can teach managers a lot. Carefully word your questions, and if you can, get help from HR.

• The United Front: Is there an easy place to stay that would help a lot of people in your group? Going to management together (for example, to ask for better temperature control in the office) is more persuasive than going alone.

• Ideas for policies: Find out if there are any model rules for dealing with menopause at work. Work with a sympathetic HR person to make one that is specific to your company's review. This will show that you are proactive and focused on finding solutions.

• The Big Picture: Small wins help get things done. It's possible that bringing fans to desks is just normal in your group. Over time, this leads to more talks with less pushback at first.

Getting Through the Complexities: When Support Groups Run Into Problems

It is important to remember that friend support isn't always easy, even though it is very helpful. For those possible bumps in the road, here's what to do:

• The Angry Nelly: Each group has one. Don't let their constant negativity get in the way of the positive outlook. Change the subject slowly by asking, "That's annoying. Does anyone know of a way to fix this?"

• Advice You Don't Want: Coworkers who mean well might give medical advice without being asked. Kindly refocus: "I appreciate the thought, but I'm focusing on what works at my desk right now."

• When a person needs help "Outgrow the Group": Sometimes, a person's problems need professional help. Have resources ready, like therapists who specialize in menopause, and say something like, "It sounds like individual therapy might be a good next step. I'd be happy to help you find resources."

• The Fizzle-Out Factor: People lose interest. Get new energy and a new purpose. Instead of crying, try to find a solution, have a guest speaker, or plan a group activity that is related to self-care during menopause.

The Effect of Ripples: More people are affected by you than you think.

If you're trying to make changes at work slowly, keep in mind that the power of your network goes beyond its members:

• The Ally Who Watches: People who are quiet and listen to your conversations might become your team's biggest fan. Show others how to be welcoming, and you'll see it happen.

• Getting new members: As word spreads that your group is a good place to be with other women, more women will naturally want to join.

• Changing the Culture: When you make it okay to talk about menopause, bring a fan to your desk, or suggest an interesting newsletter story, you break down old rules that hold everyone back.

You're not by yourself. By looking for friends, making connections, and planning how to push for change, you can change your own work life and make it possible for menopause to be a normal part of the modern workplace in the future.

Part 4: Advocating for Change

Chapter 10: Reasonable Adjustments: What to Ask For & Your Rights

Getting through menopause at work can be like getting through a trap. You know that things need to be changed, but what are your rights? What are some reasonable things you could ask your boss? This chapter talks about the idea of "reasonable adjustments" in the context of menopause. This will give you the tools to stand up for yourself and do well at work.

How to Understand Reasonable Adjustments: The Law In many countries, workers who are going through health problems, like menopause, are protected by the law. A lot of the time, these frameworks require employers to make "reasonable adjustments" to meet your needs. The most important thing is to know what "reasonable" means in your particular case.

• Know Your Rights: Find out about the job laws in your area, as well as any laws that apply to menopause and making accommodations at work. With this information, you can talk to your boss with confidence.

• The Focus on Functionality: Think about how the signs of menopause make it hard for you to do your job. Draw attention to the changes that need to be made to get you back to working normally and getting the most done.

• It's a Talk, Not a Demand: Making reasonable adjustments is a process that you and your boss work together on. To find answers that work for everyone, it's important to talk to each other openly.

Figuring Out What You Need: Common Menopause Symptoms and Possible Changes

There are many ways that the different signs of menopause can affect your work. Here is a list of common symptoms and the possible changes that could be made to them:

• Hot Flashes and Trouble Sleep: Ask for a desk fan, flexible starting times to make up for lost sleep, or a marked spot to cool off without drawing attention to yourself.

• Brain Fog and Concentration Lapses: If you're having a hard day, think about working from home, taking shorter breaks during the day to refocus, or using memory tools and note-taking apps.

• Mood Swings and Irritability: Talk about adjusting goals or workloads during times of high emotional volatility. Describe how these changes will actually help you be more productive in the long run.

• Tiredness and low stamina: Ask for ergonomic furniture to make you feel better, more breaks during the day, or the freedom to do your work at your own pace as long as you meet goals.

• Urinary Incontinence: Does your company offer clean bathrooms that are easy to get to? This is a basic need that isn't always met.

How to Write an Ask: The Art of the "Ask"

Your method can often make or break your request for changes. Here are some ways to make your point stronger:

• Tell us more: Be clear about what you need. Do some research ahead of time on possible changes and show them as options, not problems. That you said, "A desk fan would help me stay cool during hot flashes," is an example of being proactive.

• Say it in terms of prevention: Pay attention to how the changes make it easier for you to do your job and get more done. Do not think too much about the symptoms. "Flexible start times allow me to be well-rested and focused."

• Offer Alternatives: Be ready to offer a few possible changes, which will show that you're willing to work with others to find answers that work for everyone.

• Pay attention to privacy: You don't have to say details about your health problem. Just say that you're having short-term health problems that need to be fixed.

Beyond the First Request: The Conversation That Continues
As your menopause symptoms change, so might your wants. Keep the lines of conversation open with your boss:

• Set up check-ins: Set up short, regular check-ins to talk about how the changes are going and make any changes that are needed.

• Use data to help you: If the changes you make clearly make your performance better, bring this up in your follow-up talks.

• Write down everything: Write down what you asked for, the changes that were decided upon, and any follow-up talks. This is to protect you in case something goes wrong in the future.

When "reasonable" stops being reasonable: Growing worries and your rights

It's too bad that not all companies are open to the idea of reasonable adjustments. If you run into trouble, know what you can do:

• Get help from HR: It's usually the job of HR departments to make sure that the workplace is fair and that employment rules are followed. Ask them to help you advocate for your needs and give you advice.

• Collect Evidence: Write down times when not making the necessary changes hurts your work performance or makes the workplace unpleasant.

• Your lawyer: If things get tough, talking to an employment lawyer who specializes in disability or discrimination cases can give you the power to know your legal rights and possible next steps.

How Knowledge Can Help You: Resources and Groups to Back You Up

Finding trustworthy help and advice outside of work is very important, especially if you need to deal with legal issues or problems at work that are related to your requests:

• Government Resources: Labor offices or ministries that deal with equal opportunity often have a lot of information on disability rights, discrimination laws, and protections for women going through menopause at work. Check out their websites for help and tools you can download.

• Advocacy Groups for the Menopause: Many groups try to raise awareness about menopause at work and change policies that affect women going through it. On their websites, you might find toolkits, law guides, and even letter templates that you can change to talk to your boss.

• Legal Hotlines: Some groups give free or low-cost legal advice for people who are having problems at work. They can give you very useful information about how to understand the laws in your area and your rights within those laws.

• Online Support Communities: Look for sites or social media groups that you can trust that are focused on menopause and problems at work. You can share ideas, get information from other people about how to make changes that work, and get emotional support from people who are going through the same thing.

• Therapists and counsellors: If your boss's resistance is causing you a lot of mental and emotional stress, a therapist who specializes in women's health or workplace problems can help you process, plan ways to communicate, and get stronger for those tough talks.

Building Your Case: Writing Down the Problems and Effects
When people don't agree with or push back on your fair requests for changes, thorough documentation becomes your most powerful tool:

• Symptom Diary: Write down how often and how bad your menopause symptoms are, including when they happen at work (for example, brain fog during a key meeting, a hot flash during a client presentation, etc.).

• Impact Record: Write down the tasks at work that were hard for you because of unmanaged symptoms, as well as any mistakes you made, lost output, or missed deadlines. This shows that it has a real effect on how well you do your job.

• Communication Log: Write down everything you say to your boss and HR about your wishes. Write down the dates, times, what was talked about, and any deals (or lack of agreements) that were made.

Getting ready for resistance: Dealing with objections and staying strong

Get ready for possible pushback from your boss and come up with counterarguments:

• "This is only temporary, so just deal with it": "Many companies accept temporary changes for a variety of health reasons." This makes sure that important workers like me can keep doing their jobs.

• "We can't make exceptions for one person": "Proactive policies on menopause help many employees and make the workplace more welcoming." These kinds of rooms are already available at a lot of top businesses.

• "It's not fair to your coworkers": "Helping me take care of my health makes me a better team player." My improved productivity is good for the company as a whole and for my coworkers.

Know how much you're worth: When There's Enough

It's a sad fact that some companies are still stuck in old biases and might not want to change. You have to weigh the harm to your health against the good things about staying in those situations:

• Mental Health Toll: Is the constant stress of trying to get simple accommodations making you feel bad about yourself and hurting your health? Giving up your mental health for a job is never worth it.

• Looking at your options: Are there other jobs in the company where you might have a boss who is more understanding? Before doing anything dramatic, start asking around in a quiet way.

• The Plan for Getting Out: If your work setting gets bad, you should update your resume and start looking for a new job right away. Look for companies that are known for being welcoming and helping their workers at all stages of their lives.

This fight for fair housing isn't just about meeting your own needs right now. You bring about change. You can make it possible for menopause to be publicly recognized and accepted in the modern workplace by speaking up for yourself, writing down your experiences, and looking for help from outside groups.

Chapter 11: Creating a Menopause-Friendly Workplace: What Companies Can Do

Many places of work still don't talk about menopause, so people who are going through it whisper about it in the bathroom rooms or quietly deal with it. But forward-thinking businesses know that actively raising awareness and meeting the needs of menopausal employees has real benefits, such as keeping workers longer and more productive and creating a culture of genuine acceptance that attracts top talent. Let's talk about what companies can do to make sure that no woman feels like she has to choose between her job and adjusting to this normal part of life.

The Case for Supporting Menopause: Why It's Important for Business

Policies that support women going through the menopause aren't just nice things to do; they're smart business choices that have a direct effect on a company's success:

• Less absenteeism and presenteeism: Inadequate management of symptoms leads to more sick days and, even worse, presenteeism (showing up to work while sick and not doing their job), which costs companies a lot of money.

• Keep good employees: Women who are going through menopause are often at the top of their game in terms of knowledge and skills. Losing them because of a hostile work environment is a waste of ability that your company can't afford.

• Better image: Employers who have welcoming workplaces get the best workers and have a better image as places to work. This is especially important when trying to hire young people who want to work for companies that care about society.

• Higher Productivity and Well-Being: When workers feel like they can take care of their own health, they are more focused, engaged, and productive overall. This is good for everyone, not just women going through menopause.

An Approach with Multiple Parts for Building Blocks of Change

Making the workplace truly menopause-friendly takes more than a few small actions. It needs a broad plan that focuses on teaching, making practical adjustments, and building an open culture:

• Raising Awareness at All Levels: Give menopause awareness training to workers of all ages and genders, but make it a must for managers and leadership teams. To understand and be sensitive, start at the top.

• Encourage open and normal conversations about menopause in a casual setting, such as at "Lunch and Learns" or in newsletter parts that are just for that topic. Make it seem like a normal health issue instead of something that needs to be hidden.

• Adjustments that are flexible and useful: Allow for flexible work hours, the ability to control the temperature, quiet places to take breaks, and a dress code that takes into account the fact that women experience hot flashes and may gain or lose weight.

• The Power of Law: Make a policy just for menopause that covers changes, privacy, and support tools. This makes it clear what you stand for and protects the business and its employees.

Active Support: More Than Just the Basics

Companies that are really ahead of the curve will go even further to show that they care about the health and happiness of their employees at all stages of life:

• Free or low-cost health care: Look into different insurance plans that cover more treatments linked to menopause, like hormone therapy, specialist visits, and so on.

• Menopause Mentorship: Pair female workers who are going through or are close to menopause with those who are just starting to feel the symptoms, giving them advice and support.

• Benefits packages for everyone: Menopausal women often have to take on more than one caregiving job in addition to their work responsibilities. To help them, offer options like on-site child care or eldercare support.

It's important to be aware of how menopause affects people of different races, gender identities, disabilities, and socioeconomic backgrounds. Actively fight against any biases or hurdles that might be made worse.

It takes time for change to happen: Plans for Putting Things into Action

Changing deeply ingrained attitudes at work doesn't happen quickly, but small, strategic steps can help get there:

• Employee surveys: Get secret information from your employees to get a sense of the problems they're having with menopause. This helps you decide how quickly you need to act and how to tailor your policy measures.

• HR as a Leader: Give your Human Resources team the information, tools, and freedom to make choices about reasonable changes without too much red tape.

• External Partnerships: Work with experts in women's health, menopause, or support groups to give your employees training, workshops, and easy-to-find tools.

• Rejoicing in the wins: Recognize in public the good results, like higher retention rates and support from employees. This helps things move forward and fights the idea that these changes are hard.

Overcoming Problems: Dealing with Rejection and Promoting Advocacy

People who don't know better, hold on to old ideas, or are afraid of setting a bad example can sometimes fight against changes that are meant to improve the workplace. To deal with those problems, do the following:

• The "cost" stance: Add info to the counter. The much bigger cost is lost productivity, employee turnover, and a bad image as an employer who doesn't accept everyone.

• The Simple "Slippery Slope" Lie: "If we do this for menopause, everyone will want special treatment!" It's important to stress that this is about recognizing a shared medical fact, not a bunch of different people's whims.

Some men might think this is only a "women's issue" and not bother with it. Menopause-friendly workplaces are good for everyone because they boost morale, make everyone feel welcome, and draw better workers.

• Giving employees a voice: Supporters can be trained and encouraged to work as menopausal workers. It should become normal for them to talk about their experiences at work meetings, share tools, or even form a support group.

Change from the Ground Up: The Power of Employees as Champions

Support from the top down is important, but some of the most powerful changes happen naturally within the workforce. Here's how to give your workers the power to push for a more menopause-friendly workplace:

• The Informal Network: Tell workers who are going through menopause to get together and form informal support groups. This creates a place to find shared needs and plan how to advocate for them.

• Making Friends Across Identity: Women who are going through menopause shouldn't have to fight this battle by themselves. Get younger women involved who will benefit from these policies in the future, as well as guys whose partners are going through menopause and people who care about inclusion in general.

• The Proposal Approach: Give workers the freedom to write a sample policy on menopause or offer a pilot program with specific accommodations for their department. This shows that they want to find an answer.

• Success leads to more success: For example, "I negotiated flexible hours and my productivity soared!" ask workers to talk about good experiences they had because of accommodations. This shows the real benefits for the business.

Why everyone benefits from women's health

It is important to stress that companies that are friendly to women going through the menopause aren't just for women. They basically make the environment more supportive and understanding, which has many good effects:

. A culture of care: Companies that care about their workers' health and make accommodations for short-term needs show that they see them as people, not just parts of a machine. Everyone is happier about this.

• Generational Bridge: Talking about menopause breaks down barriers based on age, which helps employees at different stages of life understand each other and learn from each other, which eventually leads to more innovation and knowledge transfer.

• Taking care of all medical needs: Making it easy to talk about health problems at work makes it easier for people who are dealing with other conditions, like chronic migraines or cancer treatment, to get help.

• The Factor of Attractiveness: Millennials give more weight to companies who have policies that are welcoming to everyone. A company that supports women going through the menopause shows that it is forward-thinking and cares about its employees' health in the long run.

How the ideal workplace has changed over time

In the end, helping workers who are going through menopause is more than just helping those who are having symptoms right now. It's an important step towards getting rid of the old idea that workers should leave their personal lives, health problems, and the normal ageing process at home.

Supporting menopause knowledge, accommodations, and open communication is a step towards a truly inclusive workplace model where all employees, no matter their gender, age, or stage of life, feel valued, supported, and able to reach their full potential.

Chapter 12: Driving the Change: Advocacy at Work and Beyond

In this book, we've talked about the problems women can have when they're going through menopause while also working. This isn't a story about passive pain, though; it's a call to act. It doesn't matter if you're going through menopause yourself, are in charge of a team, or just want to make the world of work a better place. You can make it so that menopause isn't a career-ending event, but just another stage of life that workplaces understand and support.
From one person to a group: Getting people in your circle of influence to change
Protests can happen on different levels. Let's talk about how you can make a real change at work, no matter what position you hold:

• The Power of One: Break the ice, even if official rules haven't caught up yet. Make it normal to talk about menopause with a trusted coworker, ask for a fan at your desk in a sneaky way, or suggest an interesting email article. Every action breaks the rule.
• Mentorship Is Important: If you are further along in the menopause process, share how you deal with it with people who are just starting to go through it. If you're younger, be an ally, push for training in understanding, and help get rid of ageist bias.
• Managers as Agents of Change: If you are in charge of other people, you should learn about menopause, be proactive about talks about it, and be open to creative solutions. The way you lead sets the tone for everyone on your team.
• HR as Friends (Or Not): Look at Human Resources to see if they can really help change policy. Be careful if they seem unwilling to cooperate, and if you need to, think about asking higher-level leaders for help.

• Collective Strength: Are there other people at work who want to push for progress? Form an informal group in a sneaky way to share ideas, fight for resources, and help each other when talking to management.

Getting your message across: advocacy outside of work
For systemic change to happen, it needs to have an impact on a large area. Here are some ways you can join that bigger movement:

• Social media savvy: Use your accounts to share accurate information about menopause, spread the word about campaigns, or highlight companies that are making workplaces more helpful.

• Organizations that help: Find reliable non-profits that teach about and support menopause. Give them your time, your knowledge, or your money to help their work.

• Your Voice Has Power: Get in touch with your lawmakers and ask them to support laws that require job protections for women going through menopause or that make it easier for people in this stage of life to get the health care they need.

• Impact on the Industry: You belong to a work group, right? Encourage conferences to have sessions on the menopause, create a subcommittee to focus on the issue, or push for the creation of resources or guidelines that are special to the industry.

• Putting the Story to the Test: Take a look at how menopause is presented in movies and TV shows. Call out ageist tropes or damaging stereotypes, and praise the positive portrayals that help make this a normal part of life.

Conclusion: Menopause and Your Future Work Menopause is a natural part of life; it's not the end of your job.

Some people's signs are mild and easy to deal with, but others have to deal with big problems that employers have usually ignored.

Women going through menopause right now will benefit from the fight for policies that include them, the push to break down taboos, and the demand to be treated with respect and support. These things will also help women in the future.

Workplaces that are good for women going through menopause will have open and honest conversations, so employees can talk about their symptoms without feeling bad about it and get help without feeling bad about it.

• It's normal to make accommodations: People are given flexibility, temperature adjustments, and knowledge of cognitive changes proactively, not reluctantly when asked.

• Knowledge is power: All employees are taught about menopause, which builds understanding and gets rid of ageist and sexist biases.

• Women do well, not just get by: Menopausal workers don't just get through their working years; they reach their full potential and are praised for their experience and accomplishments.

You are the first person to change. If you don't suffer in silence, speak up for yourself, find allies, and push for both company-specific policies and larger societal changes, you are creating a future where menopause isn't an obstacle in a woman's career path but an accepted and supported part of a full and productive working life.

Do something: You have the power to change the future. The fight for settings that are friendly to women going through menopause isn't just about dealing with hot flashes and mood swings. For women at this natural point in their lives, it's about demanding respect, dignity, and the right to keep growing in their job. The question is: How will you help make this world what it will be? You can start making a difference right away by:

• If you are going through menopause, remember that you are not the only one. Write down your symptoms, see a doctor, put yourself first, and don't be afraid to bring it up at work, even if it seems scary at first.

As a coworker, you should learn more about menopause. Show simple kindness by giving someone a word of support, taking over for someone who is having brain fog, or speaking up for a cooler office temperature. Small acts of friendship count.

• If you're a manager, show understanding. Offer flexibility, be open to changes, and learn about the tools available to you so you can help your team members. What you do has an effect on other people.

• If you work in HR, fight for change. Learn about laws and policies that apply to women going through menopause, and work to make your company a leader in supporting all employees.

• For Everyone: Tell other people what you know. Make it normal to talk about menopause at home, with friends, and in public. Fight against old stereotypes and work to get menopause talked about in the media and in general talks about women's health.

Sample Letter Template: Contacting Your Representatives

Change often starts with making your voice heard by those in power. Here's a basic template you can adapt to email or mail to your elected officials:

Dear [Representative's Name],

I am writing as your constituent to express concern about the lack of menopause-inclusive policies and support structures for working women. Menopause is a natural biological process impacting a significant portion of the workforce, yet it remains shrouded in stigma and misunderstanding.

I urge you to support legislation that:

Mandates workplace protections for employees experiencing menopause symptoms (ex: flexible schedules, temperature regulation, etc.)

Expands access to affordable, menopause-specific healthcare resources

Promotes public awareness campaigns to combat harmful stereotypes and misinformation around menopause

Women deserve the right to thrive throughout their working lives, regardless of their age or life stage. Your leadership on this issue is crucial in creating a more just and equitable society for all.

Sincerely, [Your Name] [Your Address]

The Power of One, Multiplied

Conclusion: Menopause and Your Career Future – Embracing the Power of Menopause in the Workplace

Throughout this book, we've talked about how hard it is to deal with menopause in a world that isn't always built with women's bodies and life cycles in mind. This is not a story of loss; it's a story of change. Even though menopause can be hard, it can also be a chance: a chance to take back our stories, create new ways of working, and release a strong group of experienced women who refuse to be ignored or pushed to the side.

Imagine working in a place where: • Women in their 40s and 50s are valued assets: Instead of ageist stereotypes that focus on getting worse, businesses know that women going through menopause are at the top of their game when it comes to experience, knowledge, and strategic thinking.

• Being wise is admired, not feared: women who are going through menopause are sought after as leaders, teachers, and new ideas. Their unique points of view, which come from having lived and worked in different situations, are very helpful to the companies they work for.

• Self-advocacy is the norm: women are free to be open about their needs, ask for accommodations without feeling bad about it, and put their health first as a must if they want to keep working. • Being flexible is essential: jobs are made to fit people's wants, not old, rigid structures. Flexible hours, controlling the temperature, and being able to talk openly about changes in mental state are the norm, not the exception.

• Group power leads to systemic change: What started as a few individual voices has grown into a movement calling for big changes in policies, healthcare for everyone, and a big change in how society understands, talks about, and supports the wide range of working experiences women have.

This thought of the future isn't just idealistic; it's actually possible.

With hard work, knowledge, and the planned actions we've talked about in this book, we can slowly but surely break down hurtful stereotypes and create a workplace where women can thrive during the life-changing journey of menopause, not just survive it.

Helpful and empowering resources for you

This book is just the start of your journey. To help you keep learning, speaking out, and getting the help you need, here are some places to start:

• Groups that fight for menopause: Find trustworthy non-profits that want to raise awareness, change laws, and help the community. On their websites, you can often grab toolkits, fact sheets, and links to support groups in your area.

• Therapists and counsellors: Look for women's health experts, especially therapists who know how to help women with the physical and mental health problems that come with menopause. Aside from the workplace, they can offer personalized tactics and help.

• Online communities and forums: The power of having the same experience is very strong. Find internet forums or social media groups that you can trust that are focused on work and menopause. In a group of people who really get it, you can share tips, vent your frustrations, and get ideas.

• Resources for the government: Find out if the labor departments in your state, country, or other relevant organizations have websites that talk about women's health, disability rights, or age discrimination in the workplace. These often have useful information in them that can help you understand your legal rights.

Why strategic advocacy is important: safety, privacy, and effect

Sharing your story can be very powerful, but you need to make sure you do it in a way that puts your safety and well-being first. Not every workplace is open to change, and unfortunately, speaking out can sometimes lead to discrimination or bad reactions. Here's how to keep up strategic advocacy while keeping your job risks to a minimum:

• Look at your environment. Is the culture of your job generally open to new ideas? Are there helpful people in power roles that you can quietly talk to? Before you choose a level of openness, you need to be honest about your work setting.

• Strength in Numbers: If openly advocating feels dangerous, is there a way to get together with other women who feel the same way and talk to

HR or management as a group? Anonymized surveys that record common problems can be a better first step in some cases.

• Know what rights you have: Find out about your area's anti-discrimination rules and any employment protections that may apply to the menopause. Knowing this gives you power over your decisions, even if you never have to use your legal rights.

• Keep track of things: Keep a secret record of the problems you're having at work because of menopause. Write down specific events, your requests for help, and whether or not they were met. These steps will help you build a case if you have problems at work next time.

Take care of your health first: If the people you work with become openly hostile because of your advocacy, your physical and mental health should come first. Start looking for other jobs in a sneaky way, and remember that no job is worth giving up your pride or putting yourself in serious danger for.

The fight for progress goes on.

The work of making businesses truly menopause-friendly is still going on. It could have both happy times of success and frustrating setbacks. Remember that even small things like making talks seem normal, asking for small changes, or teaching others in a subtle way have an impact that goes far beyond your own workspace.

This book is meant to give you the information, strategies, and support network you need to deal with the unique problems that

menopause can bring up in your job. It's meant to get you to speak up for yourself and join a larger movement that changes how we see, talk about, and help women of all ages as they go through every stage of their working lives.

The future of work is open to everyone, caring, and made to accommodate the wide range of human experiences. It will not be hard to go through menopause; it will be seen as a normal part of life and be supported. Let's work together to make that idea come true.